PHOSPHATIDYLSERINE

The Comprehensive Guide to Boost
Brain Function, Combat Stress, and
Enhance Learning for Peak
Performance and Overall Well-being

SAMANTHA ZYLAR

Contents

CHAPTER ONE

Overview

One essential phospholipids that is essential to many bodily functions in humans is phosphatidylserine or PS. High amounts of this naturally occurring lipid are present in cell membranes, especially in the brain.

The importance of phosphatidylserine for memory retention, cognitive function, and general brain health is well known. It is also acknowledged for its possible therapeutic uses in treating a variety of illnesses, such as age-related cognitive decline and stress reduction.

We will examine the structure, function, dietary sources, and significance of phosphatidylserine in sustaining brain health and general well-being as we delve into this complex issue. Phosphatidylserine is important for the scientific and medical communities, but it's also important for anyone trying to improve their mental health and cognitive function.

Phosphatidylserine is a prime example of the complex nature of biochemical substances and their significant influence on our day-to-day existence due to its complicated involvement in maintaining brain health and cell membrane integrity.

Understanding phosphatidylserine's structural and functional characteristics as well as its useful uses in improving cognitive function and quality of life is crucial to understanding the substance's relevance.

What Phosphatidylserine Is All About

All living things have cell membranes that include phospholipids called phosphatidylserine, or PS for short. The brain has the highest concentration of PS in the body. This vital substance is directly linked to cognitive function and general brain health, and it is crucial to many physiological functions.

What Is Phosphatidylserine?

One kind of phospholipids—a class of chemicals essential to cell membranes—is phosphatidylserine. It is a fatty material made up of a serine molecule, two fatty acid chains, a phosphate group, and a glycerol backbone. Because of its special makeup, it can be found in the inner leaflet of the cell membrane, where it is essential for preserving the fluidity and integrity of these membranes.

Phosphatidylserine is involved in signaling, membrane transport, and neurotransmitter release, in addition to its structural involvement in cell membranes. Notably, it is necessary for intercellular contacts because it provides a platform for proteins that are in charge of cell signaling and communication.

It's Significance For Mental Wellness

1. Neurotransmitter Regulation: The correct action of neurotransmitters depends on phosphatidylserine. Chemicals called neurotransmitters are responsible for sending messages

throughout the brain, and their effectiveness depends on the integrity of cell membranes. In order to ensure effective communication between neurons, phosphatidylserine aids in maintaining the fluidity of these membranes. Consequently, this directly affects memory, mood control, and cognitive processes.

2. PS also has an impact on the defense of neurons against harm. It functions as an antioxidant, assisting in the reduction of oxidative stress and inflammation's detrimental effects on the brain. Phosphatidylserine prolongs the lifespan and general health of neurons by lowering the risk of damage to brain cells.

3. Enhancement of Cognitive Function: Phosphatidylserine supplements appear to have a beneficial effect on cognitive function. Its ability to enhance learning, memory, and attention has been researched. It might also benefit people who are experiencing cognitive impairment or age-related cognitive decline.

4. Stress reaction: Research indicates that phosphatidylserine contributes to the body's stress reaction. It can assist in controlling the release of stress hormones like cortisol, which, when persistently high, can have negative effects on brain function. By modulating the stress reaction, PS

could promote mental health in general.

5.   Neurological   Disorders: Phosphatidylserine supplementation may be helpful in treating some neurological conditions, including attention deficit hyperactivity disorder (ADHD) and Alzheimer's disease, according to some research. The potential neuroprotective and cognitive-enhancing effects of PS seem encouraging, notwithstanding the need for additional investigation.

In summary, phosphatidylserine is an essential part of cell membranes, particularly in the brain, where it is critical for preserving mental health and cognitive function. Its importance in promoting mental health is highlighted by its role in neurotransmitter modulation, neuronal protection, and cognitive enhancement. Although a healthy diet can provide it, there are supplements available for individuals looking to improve the health of their brains or deal with certain cognitive issues. In the field of neuroscience and brain health, phosphatidylserine is still an interesting and important component as additional study reveals its possible advantages.

The Phosphatidylserine Story

PS, or phosphatidylserine, is a vital phospholipid that is involved in many different physiological functions in the human body. Its history is replete with discoveries and in-depth studies that have revealed its primary purposes.

Let us examine the historical background of phosphatidylserine, emphasizing its discovery and significant turning points in our comprehension of its importance.

Investigation And Initial Research

The Swiss biologist Ernst Schülen and his associates found and isolated phosphatidylserine for the first time in 1942. This phospholipid was first discovered in the brain tissue of cows. The scientific investigation of PS and its importance in biological systems commenced with this discovery.

Phosphatidylserine structural and chemical characteristics, as well as its function as a component of cell membranes, were the main subjects of early research. Its importance as a constituent of the lipid bilayer, the building block of cell membranes, was realized by scientists. This basic knowledge prepared the way for additional research on PS's roles in cell biology and physiology.

Understanding Milestones

1. Membrane Structure: The fluid mosaic model of cell membranes was better understood in the 1950s and 60s because of studies on phospholipids such as PS. PS has been identified as a critical component in preserving the fluidity and integrity of the membrane, which is necessary for a number of biological functions, including signal transduction and the movement of molecules across the cell membrane.

2. Blood Clotting: In the 1970s, scientists made great strides toward

clarifying PS's function in blood coagulation. It was discovered that exposure to PS on the surface of blood cells, including platelets, is essential for the coagulation cascade and aids in the creation of blood clots.

3. Neurological and Cognitive performance: Phosphatidylserine effects on brain health and cognitive performance were first studied by researchers in the 1980s and 1990s.

Research suggests that PS supplementation might improve cognitive function, memory, and attention. As a result, PS-based supplements were created.

4. Aging and Stress Management: Phosphatidylserine may help with stress management and aging, according to research conducted in the last few decades. According to studies, PS may improve cognitive performance in elderly persons and lessen the harmful effects of stress on the body.

5. Clinical Uses: Phosphatidylserine is now being used in clinical settings, mostly for Alzheimer's and other cognitive problems.

To fully understand its therapeutic potential in different neurological diseases, research is still ongoing.

Phosphatidylserine history demonstrates the continuous investigation into the functions and uses of this phospholipid in human biology and health. Since its first discovery in the 1940s, PS has attracted scientific attention and innovation, and its importance in neurology, psychology, and medicine has only grown.

CHAPTER TWO

The Function Of Phosphatidylserine In Biology

One important phospholipid that is involved in many different biological processes in the human body is phosphatidylserine or PS. Its involvement in neurotransmitter function, presence in cell membranes, and control over apoptosis underscore its importance in preserving general physiological processes.

1. Cell Membrane Structure:

One of the main phospholipids that make up cell

membranes is phosphatidylserine. It supports the lipid bilayer's fluidity and structural integrity. Because PS has a negatively charged serine group—which is necessary for healthy membrane function—it differs from other phospholipids. Its location inside the lipid bilayer is essential for preserving the fluidity and stability of the membrane as well as for controlling the actions of essential membrane proteins. Moreover, PS has the ability to function as a signaling molecule, promoting connections with other proteins and signaling pathways that influence how cells react to different stimuli. It is especially prevalent in the inner leaflet of the plasma membrane, where phagocytic cells use it as an "eat-me" signal to facilitate the removal of apoptotic cells.

2. Role In The Function Of Neurotransmitters:

Phosphatidylserine also has a role in the function of neurotransmitters, especially in the central nervous system. It acts as a precursor to acetylcholine, one of the neurotransmitters. Acetylcholine is necessary for neurons to send information across synapses, which is why PS is important for cognitive processes like memory and learning. Sufficient levels of PS are essential for preserving a balanced neurotransmitter system, and research indicates that supplementing with PS may improve cognitive function, particularly in older adults.

3. Apoptosis:

Phosphatidylserine is essential for the tightly controlled process of programmed cell death known as apoptosis. Cells go through a sequence of actions during apoptosis that culminates in their deliberate self-destruction. The exposure of PS on the surface of their outer membrane, which alerts macrophages and other phagocytic cells to identify and devour the dying cell, is one of the distinguishing characteristics of apoptotic cells. This helps to maintain tissue homeostasis by preventing the leakage of hazardous cellular contents into the surrounding tissue. The strictly controlled exposure of PS during apoptosis is important for immunological tolerance and the avoidance of autoimmune reactions.

To summarize, phosphatidylserine is a complex phospholipid that plays an essential part in neurotransmitter function, cell membrane structure, and apoptosis regulation. Its involvement in these processes is essential for preserving the structural integrity of tissues and cells, promoting intercellular communication within the nervous system, and guaranteeing the appropriate removal of harmed or dying cells. Phosphatidylserine's biological role highlights the significance of this essential nutrient in preserving general health and physiological processes.

Phosphatidylserine In Mental Processes

A phospholipid called phosphatidylserine (PS) is a necessary constituent of cell membranes, especially those of brain cells. It is essential for several facets of cognitive function, including mood and stress reduction, focus and attention span improvement, and memory improvement. Here's a closer look at the ways in which phosphatidylserine affects various mental processes:

1. Memory Enhancement: Many studies have looked into the possibility of phosphatidylserine to improve memory. It is thought to aid memory in a number of ways:

• Enhanced neural communication: Phosphatidylserine facilitates effective signal transmission between brain cells by maintaining the fluidity and integrity of cell membranes. This could improve the mechanisms via which memories are created and retrieved.

• Neuroprotective effects: It demonstrates neuroprotective qualities, which might enhance memory retention and prevent brain cells from harm over the long run.

• Increased release of acetylcholine: Acetylcholine is a neurotransmitter that is essential for learning and memory. Acetylcholine release in the brain may be enhanced by phosphatidylserine, and this may have a beneficial effect on memory performance.

2. Potential Enhancement:

Phosphatidylserine has the potential to enhance attention and focus in multiple ways.

• Improved cell membrane integrity: Phosphatidylserine can support the maintenance of brain cells' optimal functioning, which is necessary for focus and attention, by protecting the integrity of neuronal cell membranes.

• Lower cortisol levels: Excessive cortisol levels, which are frequently linked to stress, can impair concentration and focus. It has been demonstrated that phosphatidylserine helps control cortisol levels, which may improve cognitive function.

3. Mood And Stress Management:

Phosphatidylserine possible contribution to mood and stress management has also drawn attention.

• Stress reduction: By inhibiting the release of the stress hormone cortisol, phosphatidylserine may help lessen the body's reaction to stress. An increase in mood and emotional health may arise from this.

• Enhanced neurotransmitter balance: Phosphatidylserine improves the balance of numerous neurotransmitters, including serotonin, dopamine, and norepinephrine, which play essential roles in mood regulation. This balance can contribute to increased emotional stability.

In conclusion, phosphatidylserine is a phospholipid that is essential for a number of cognitive processes, such as mood and stress reduction, concentration and attention, and memory improvement. It affects neurotransmitter balance, stress hormone control, and cell membrane integrity to produce these effects. Phosphatidylserine is therefore frequently seen as a beneficial supplement for people wishing to support and improve their mental and emotional health. But before adding any supplement to your regimen, especially if you have underlying medical concerns or are on other medications, it is imperative that you speak with a healthcare provider.

Sources Of Phosphatidylserine In Nature

One important phospholipid that is vital to preserving the integrity and functionality of cell membranes, especially those in the brain, is phosphatidylserine, or PS. It participates in a number of biological functions, such as neurotransmitter release, cell-to-cell communication, and signal transduction. Even while the body can produce some PS, it's usually best to get it from food or supplements. This is a summary of phosphatidylserine's natural sources, which include foods high in PS, dietary supplements, and appropriate amounts.

Foods High In Serine Phosphate:

1. Organ Meats: The liver is one of the most abundant natural sources of PS. Specifically, cow brains have remarkably high PS levels.

2. Fatty Fish: Fish with intermediate PS levels include mackerel and herring. Adding these fish to your diet can increase your PS consumption.

3. White Beans: Plant-based sources of PS include kidney beans, soybeans, and white beans. To encourage the consumption of PS, they offer a vegetarian variant.

4. Dairy items: Cheese and cow's milk are two examples of dairy items that may contain trace quantities of PS. Because whole milk has more fat than skim milk, it contains more PS.

5. Phosphatidylserine is found in sunflower lecithin, which is

frequently employed as an emulsifier in a variety of food products.

Dietary Supplements:

Sunflower or soy lecithin is the primary source of phosphatidylserine, which is found in supplements. Supplements like these can be a useful method to increase your PS intake, particularly if you prefer a more controlled dosage or have dietary constraints. They are frequently used to boost memory and cognitive function, especially in older persons, and come in a variety of forms, including powders and capsules.

Effective Doses: Depending on a person's requirements, age, and health, there are several possible phosphatidylserine dosages. Generally speaking, it is advised to speak with a healthcare provider before beginning any supplementation. Nonetheless, the following broad principles apply:

1. Cognitive Enhancement: A typical dosage range for PS is 100–300 mg daily in order to support cognitive function and increase memory.

2. Stress Reduction: Higher doses (300–600 mg daily) may be useful, according to some research, in lowering cortisol levels and reducing

stress, especially for athletes and people with high-stress lives.

3. ADHD and Cognitive Decline: Subjects with age-related cognitive decline or attention deficit hyperactivity disorder (ADHD) have received 200–400 mg of PS daily in certain clinical trials.

4. Activity Performance: To lessen stress brought on by activity and enhance recuperation, athletes may find that taking 300–800 mg of PS daily is beneficial.

It's critical to keep an eye on how your body reacts to phosphatidylserine and modify the dosage as necessary. Even though it's usually regarded as harmless, side effects can happen, such as stomach problems and insomnia occasionally. As with any supplement, it's best to see a healthcare professional to figure out the right dosage and make sure it won't have any unfavorable interactions with other prescriptions or medical problems.

CHAPTER THREE

Phosphatidylserine In Therapeutic Contexts

A phospholipid substance called phosphatidylserine (PS) is essential to the composition and operation of cell membranes, especially those of brain cells. Although it can be found in trace levels in a variety of foods, including soy, it can also be purchased as a nutritional supplement. Potential clinical uses for phosphatidylserine have drawn interest, especially in the fields of Alzheimer's disease and dementia,

ADHD, cognitive disorders, and stress and anxiety management.

1. Alzheimer's Disease And Dementia:

Phosphatidylserine has demonstrated potential as a treatment option for people suffering from dementia, including Alzheimer's disease. Studies indicate that it could potentially enhance memory and cognitive abilities while also delaying the onset of cognitive deterioration. By improving neurotransmitter function and encouraging the production of acetylcholine, a neurotransmitter essential for memory and learning, PS is thought to improve brain health.

Phosphatidylserine supplementation may be helpful in the early stages of Alzheimer's disease and in treating memory-related problems in older persons, while further research is required.

2. ADHD And Other Cognitive Disorders:

Problems with focus, attention, and impulse control are common features of attention-deficit/hyperactivity disorder (ADHD) and other cognitive disorders. It has been investigated whether phosphatidylserine could be used as an additional therapy for people with ADHD and other cognitive impairments.

Supplementing with PS may improve cognitive performance, especially in the domains of impulse control, attention, and focus, according to certain research. It is believed to function by promoting the brain's dopamine and norepinephrine receptor sites, which are important in controlling focus and attention.

3. Anxiety And Stress:

The possible benefits of phosphatidylserine in reducing anxiety and stress have also been studied. Elevated levels of the stress hormone cortisol, which can have a negative impact on general well-being and cognitive performance, are a result of chronic stress. By assisting in the regulation of cortisol levels, phosphatidylserine may lessen the negative effects of stress on the body and mind. It is thought to uplift the adrenal glands and support a more balanced level of cortisol, both of which can lead to a calmer mental state and enhanced cognitive function.

Phosphatidylserine supplements are utilized in clinical practice for these purposes, with differing degrees of success. It's crucial to remember that, even if certain studies have produced encouraging results, additional investigation is required to confirm the treatment's efficacy and safety in various clinical contexts.

Furthermore, each person may require a different quantity and length of supplementation; therefore speaking with a healthcare provider is advised before beginning any supplementation program, particularly for the treatment of particular medical issues.

Phosphatidylserine is a natural substance that shows promise for use in medicine, especially when it comes to treating cognitive problems, Alzheimer's disease, ADHD, stress, and anxiety. Its efficacy and ideal application in these domains will be further clarified by ongoing study and clinical trials.

Security And Possible Adverse Reactions

The body naturally produces phosphatidylserine (PS), which is a phospholipid that is abundant in brain cells and found in cell membranes throughout the body. Its possible ability to improve memory and cognition has drawn interest. Although it is usually regarded as safe when taken as prescribed, there are a few crucial factors to take into account when using it long-term, including possible hazards, side effects, precautions, and interactions with other medications.

Security And Possible Adverse Reactions:

1. Generally Recognized as Safe (GRAS): The United States has designated phosphatidylserine as Generally Recognized as Safe. FDA when taken in accordance with dosage recommendations. It is safe for most people to take and seldom causes negative side effects.

2. Mild Side Effects: When taking phosphatidylserine, some people may have mild gastrointestinal symptoms like diarrhea or upset stomach. Most of the time, these adverse effects are dose-dependent and temporary.

3. Allergies: While they are uncommon, allergic responses to PS might happen. In the event that you develop symptoms such as rash, swelling, itching, or trouble breathing, stop using the product and visit a doctor.

Risks And Safety Measures:

1. Pregnancy and Breastfeeding: Not much research has been done on the safety of phosphatidylserine during pregnancy and nursing. It is best for those who are breastfeeding or pregnant to speak with a healthcare

provider before taking PS supplements.

2. Medical Conditions: Before taking phosphatidylserine, see your doctor if you have any underlying medical conditions, particularly bleeding disorders.

PS may interfere with blood coagulation, so people who have bleeding issues should be cautious.

Interactions Between Drugs:

1. Anticoagulants and Antiplatelet Drugs: Interactions between phosphatidylserine and anticoagulants

(blood thinners) like aspirin or warfarin are possible. It is important to let your healthcare provider know if you are taking these medications because they may increase your risk of bleeding.

2.   Cholinergic   drugs: Phosphatidylserine may interact with certain   drugs,   such   as acetylcholinesterase inhibitors used to treat Alzheimer's disease.

Theoretically, combining them could increase cholinergic activity and cause adverse symptoms including nausea, vomiting, or diarrhea.

3. Medication for Blood Pressure: PS may have the ability to drop blood

pressure, which may interfere with drugs intended to treat hypertension. If you intend to utilize phosphatidylserine while taking blood pressure medicine, speak with a healthcare provider beforehand.

Considerations For Long-Term Use:

1. Tolerance and Efficacy: According to certain research, Phosphatidylserine's ability to improve cognition may wear off after prolonged use. To sustain efficacy, regular breaks or cycling might be taken into consideration.

2. Dosing: Recommendations for long-term use should be followed. Overuse raises the possibility of drug interactions and negative consequences.

3. Frequent Monitoring: It is recommended to periodically meet with a healthcare provider for health evaluations and to monitor any potential side effects if you plan to use phosphatidylserine for an extended period of time.

In summary, phosphatidylserine is typically safe when used as prescribed; nevertheless, people with certain medical conditions and those on particular drugs should exercise caution. Before beginning any new supplement regimen, especially if you have underlying health concerns or want to use it for an extended period of time, it is imperative that you speak with a healthcare expert. Always take prescription medications as directed, and watch out for any negative side effects.

Phosphatidylserine Future

A phospholipid called phosphatidylserine is an essential constituent of cell membranes, especially those in the brain. Phosphatidylserine has been the subject of research for many years, and interest in it has grown due to its possible advantages for mood, stress reduction, and cognitive health. Phosphatidylserine research has a number of exciting new directions and areas to investigate in the future.

1. Improvement Of Cognitive Function And Neuroprotection:

Phosphatidylserine's effects on cognitive function and neuroprotection are likely to be further explored in future studies. Research may examine its function in improving learning, memory, and general brain health.

To optimize phosphatidylserine's impact on cognition, research into how it interacts with other substances or nutrients may provide novel insights.

2. Mood And Stress Management: By controlling the body's reaction to the stress hormone cortisol, phosphatidylserine has demonstrated the potential to lower stress and elevate mood.

Subsequent investigations could concentrate on comprehending the exact mechanisms and pathways involved in this process, which could result in the creation of innovative treatments for ailments linked to stress and mood disorders.

3. Physical Health And Sports Performance:

Phosphatidylserine has been researched in relation to sports performance, specifically in terms of lowering stress brought on by exercise and enhancing recuperation.

Its impact on physical health, inflammation reduction, and muscle function may be further studied. Enhancements in supplement compositions, amounts, and modes of administration may maximize their application within the sports community.

4. Age-Related Cognitive Decline And Neurodegenerative Disorders:

As the population ages, age-related cognitive decline and neurodegenerative disorders such as Alzheimer's are becoming more common.

Subsequent research endeavors may investigate the potential of phosphatidylserine to decelerate the advancement of such ailments or even function as a prophylactic strategy. In this context, studies may also concentrate on the synergistic effects of phosphatidylserine with other substances or lifestyle variables.

5. Novel Delivery Methods And Combinations:

To improve Phosphatidylserine's bioavailability, researchers may use novel delivery methods such as liposomal formulations or nanoparticles. Furthermore, phosphatidylserine may be more beneficial for products or interventions when combined with other nutrients or substances that promote brain health and cognitive performance.

6. Phosphatidylserine Efficacy:

Phosphatidylserine study may investigate how a person's genetics, lifestyle, and health state affect how well they respond to supplements, as the field of personalized medicine continues to develop. Customizing advice according to these variables may improve phosphatidylserine's efficacy for every individual.

7. Safety And Long-Term Effects:

Further investigation is

required to evaluate the possible adverse effects and long-term safety of supplementing with phosphatidylserine. It will be essential to comprehend any drug interactions or contraindications before implementing this widely.

Phosphatidylserine research has a bright future ahead of it, with an emphasis on physical health, mental clarity, mood regulation, and creative delivery methods.

As our knowledge of this substance expands, it is probably going to become increasingly important in promoting human health and wellness in a number of ways, opening up new avenues for boosting cognitive function and general quality of life.

Conclusion

To sum up, phosphatidylserine, or PS is an amazing phospholipid that has significant effects on cognitive function and brain health. We have covered its vital function in the brain, its possible advantages, and its importance in fostering mental health throughout this conversation.

Synopsis Of Major Findings

1. Phospholipid in Brain Structure: Particularly in brain cells,

phosphatidylserine plays a critical role in cell membranes. It is crucial for preserving the fluidity and integrity of membranes, which affects cell signaling and brain function as a whole.

2. Enhancement of Cognitive Function: Studies indicate that taking PS supplements may improve cognitive functions like memory, focus, and general cognitive function. This has attracted a lot of attention, especially when considering aging and cognitive decline.

3. Stress Reduction: PS has been linked to lessening the damaging effects of stress on the nervous

system. It can lessen the damaging effects of ongoing stress on cognitive function by adjusting the body's stress response.

4. Neuroprotective Properties: PS appears to be a promising agent for protecting neurons. It could be able to stop neurodegenerative disorders like Alzheimer's from getting worse or at least slow them down.

5. Safety and Dosage: When used in accordance with suggested dosages, PS supplements are typically safe for the majority of people. It's crucial to speak with a medical expert to find out the right dosage for your unique requirements.

6. Sources of Phosphatidylserine: Although several meals contain trace levels of PS, many people use supplements to make sure their consumption is sufficient. PS supplements come in a number of forms, such as powders and pills.

Promotion Of Brain Health

It's intriguing to investigate the potential benefits of phosphatidylserine on brain health in general, especially in light of the optimistic research results. PS is an intriguing option to think about, whether your goal is to preserve cognitive function as you age or to improve your mental clarity temporarily.

If you're experiencing high levels of stress, incorporating PS into your daily routine may be especially helpful since it may help protect your brain from the damaging consequences of ongoing stress. In the same way that we emphasize physical health through exercise and a balanced diet, it is crucial to acknowledge the significance of proactive actions for brain health.

Moreover, as this field of study develops, we might find many more applications for PS that improve brain function and well-being. The most important lesson to learn from this is that we can continue to strengthen and care for our brain health throughout our lives.

For anyone looking to maximize cognitive function and protect the long-term health of their brain, it is an appealing option due to its wide range of advantages and comparatively low-risk profile. Before incorporating any dietary supplement into your wellness routine, as with any other, it is best to speak with a healthcare provider to be sure it meets your unique needs and health goals.